Diets Suck!

Diets Suck! How I Lost Weight Without Giving Up Doughnuts
by Julien McArdle.

Published by McArdle Publications. Printed by Lulu.com.
ISBN 978-0-9812642-2-6

The information contained within this work relates the experiences of the author and is for entertainment purposes only. This book is not intended as a reference of any sort. The author is not a medical professional nor has any expertise in the field. The parties behind this book, including the author, publisher, and printer, are not liable for any outcomes arising from the information presented in this book. Please consult a medical professional for health matters.

To Jay

Table of Contents

Introduction

S tories like mine seem to be a dime a dozen. I struggled with weight all my life, enduring years of bullying in school over my size. Then the excess pounds came off and I entered adulthood a slender individual.

Nevertheless, I still saw myself as fat. The verbal abuse I endured as a child had taken its toll and completely warped my self-image. It would only be much later that I would come to recognize this distortion, and later yet that I'd sever the mental pairing of beauty with the numbers on a scale.

Following university, my weight exploded. I attempted a number of unhealthy approaches to bring it under control, but they never worked. I'd lose thirty pounds, then gain fifty. I became obese.

Comments about my weight resumed, this time under the pretence of concern from family and friends. It was as if they assumed that my size was as a result of my inability to see myself in a mirror, or to comprehend the ceaseless remarks made by the world around me. I found that time had not made these comments hurt any less.

Good things did come to happen, however. I met my boyfriend, who loved me as I was and never wavered in his support. He helped me appreciate myself and work towards overcoming the distorted view of my body that had etched its way into my psyche. I also abandoned weight loss for the sake of assimilating into a society obsessed with slim waist-lines. Henceforth, any pursuit of the matter would purely be for health reasons.

This mental shift away from vanity removed my need for instant results. It also reduced my concerns with occasionally gaining back weight. I took a steady long-term approach and gave myself two years to lose fifty pounds.

The strategy worked. I ended up losing the weight and keeping it off. I did it not through food deprivation but through subtle changes to my eating habits. The idea being that very small tweaks would add up over time.

As this book's namesake suggests, I still eat doughnuts. I neither diet nor have a need for cheat days. I don't ever starve myself and have come to manage binging. In the following pages, I'll detail how I pulled it all off.

Overview

A Note for Professional Dieters

The approach discussed in this book can be summarized as calorie counting with a twist. Rather than tracking calories to set hard restrictions on daily consumption, as is typically the case, it is used as a learning tool. There is no micro-budgeting calories or paying heed to carbohydrates, fat content, and other indicators.

When I started this weight loss journey, I kept a food journal to find out how much I was consuming calorie-wise. As it turns out, I was taking in on average 500 to 1000 calories more than was recommended for my body type. To my surprise, it wasn't my main meals that made the bulk of these so much as the snacks in-between.

I set a daily calorie threshold. When I exceeded it, I told myself to ask *why* I had surpassed it. Usually, there was a few causes. Perhaps it was the chips I mindlessly ate while watching a movie at home, or the combination of eating a big meal at a restaurant along with a treat from the ice cream parlour. Using this information, I then formulated strategies that I could employ to reduce the footprint the next time while feeling as full. For instance, by mixing up the chips with something less calorie-intensive while watching that film.

The important point is that depriving myself of food was never an option. Instead, I made subtle changes to my food-related decisions, which then reduced the amount of calories I ingested. The savings weren't anything drastic, and that was fine: I was in this for the long-run.

I see this approach as counter to fad diets, those celebrity-backed crazes that capitalize on insecurities and promise significant weight loss in a matter of weeks. I wanted my weight loss to last me a life time, and I only saw that as possible if the alterations I made my eating habits did not tamper with my love of food.

Fad Diets Suck

Despite being rooted in the Greek word *diata* meaning *the way of life*, diets have become synonymous with the impermanent. The type of regimens advertised by late-night television and B-list celebrities suggest what is tantamount to temporary starvation as the means to make those pounds disappear.

The problem arises when the untenable bout of food deprivation inevitably comes to an end and there's a reversion to old eating habits. It was those behaviours that caused the weight gain that triggered the initial call to diet, and so the lost pounds all come flying back. A yo-yo is often used to analogize the gaining and losing weight that is emblematic of this cycle. It was following the end of my last tryst with such a diet that I jumped into obesity.

Finally realizing the insanity of subjugating myself to this never-ending cycle, I put an end to it and completely changed my approach. I would now make minor tweaks to my eating habits; subtle changes I could and would carry with me for life. There would be no denying cheesecakes, pasta, or anything else I enjoyed. I anticipated the weight loss attributed to this approach would be slow. I gave myself two years to achieve my target weight.

Progress was much faster than anticipated. I reached my goal of losing fifty pounds a little over a year after I had begun. I revised my target and lost ten more.

It was important that this did not become a chore. Key to this was to never feel hungry. I ate lots, but made small alterations to what I would choose to eat when a pang hit me. Thus a snack coming home from work went from bread and cheese to lots of vegetables and cereal. Or I *would* have bread and cheese – as long as I was aware of what went in my body.

Hello Calories

The first step on my path to weight loss was to become aware of how many calories I ingested. At its core, calories are a measure of the energy used by our bodies to function. Consume too much, and the excess energy is converted into fat that is stored by the body for later use. Consume too little, and the body's ability to operate properly is compromised with potentially lethal consequences.

A typical person requires about 2,000 calories each day. That said, this figure varies greatly depending on factors such as the individual's sex, age, weight, and how much exercise they do. After consulting a number of on-line resources, I found that I should have been consuming 2,200 calories. My actual intake was closer to the 2,500 – 3,500 mark.

To illustrate the impact of this excess, consuming an extra 250 calories a day, or a little less than the average chocolate bar, would have been enough to cause gains of a pound every two weeks.

All was not lost, however. As the example of the chocolate bar also shows, making small changes – such as occasionally substituting the said chocolate delicacy with a different snack – resulted in very tangible changes.

Despite the emphasis on reducing calories, it's important to re-iterate that they are an essential part of everyday living and the point is certainly not to eliminate them.

It's also worthy to note that the calorie content of food is unrelated to its nutritional value. Just because something has fewer calories does not necessarily mean it's healthy. Likewise, calorie-rich foods such as nuts can be very nutritious. For such items, the emphasis is moderation, not avoidance.

My awareness of calories was not for the establishment of hard limits as suggested by some diets. Rather, this information was to figure out *why* I exceeded my recommended daily value of 2,200 calories, and what I could do the next time round to avoid a repeat.

This approach started a positive feedback loop. As I enacted strategies to help me avoid going over my recommended daily caloric intake, my weight came down. As it dropped, so too did the recommended daily value.

Food Journal

Following my awareness to the concept of calories, the next thing I did was to keep a food journal. Either throughout the day or at its conclusion, I would note down what I ate and how many calories were in it.

```
Breakfast
140 cal – 2 Eggs
150 cal – Toast
300 cal – Sausage
 30 cal – Ketchup

Lunch
 80 cal – Deli Meat
100 cal – Wrap
510 cal – Nuts
150 cal – Soda
```

One of the first things I noticed was that there were a few items, usually not among the big meals of the day, that were responsible for a disproportionate amount of calories. A single snack, depending on what it was, could have more calories than my breakfast or lunch.

Out of this and other realizations came tricks to balance the distribution of calories and reduce their overall count without feeling hungry. I detail them in the next section, *Strategies*.

Learning Portions

A big part of my weight-loss was to be aware of how many calories were in what I ate. One of the realizations coming out of keeping the food journal was that my concept of what constituted a portion was really off. I often thought portions were bigger than they actually were.

I started to look at nutritional labels, and through the use of measuring cups and mental guesswork, determined how much was a portion of any given product. If I bought three pounds worth of apples, and I got thirteen apples of roughly the same size, then a simple division would get me an estimate of its weight. From that, I would find out how many calories there was per apple. Same with packaged meats. Investing in a food scale would have probably saved me some time.

This new-found awareness with regards to portions altered my decision making process. For instance, I found myself inadvertently tweaking proportions in my meals (*Proportioning Meals*, page 37) to maximize food enjoyment and intake while minimizing calories.

In cases where calorie information was immediately unavailable, such as when the product came from a fast food joint, I'd consult the company's website for nutritional information. If their website did not have that information, I would guess the calorie content by finding the nutritional data for similar products.

Culinary Exploration

The purpose of keeping a food journal was that simply becoming aware of the caloric cost of what I consumed altered my decision making process with food. Not in a very substantive way, but enough to make a positive difference over the long run.

Another means by which I gained this sense of awareness was by making some of the sweets I enjoyed – chocolate cookies and cheesecake for instance. I wouldn't do these from a mix but from scratch. Such efforts usually solicited a sense of surprise as I learnt just how much sugar, butter, and cream cheese made some of my staples. I've included some of the items in the following table.

Consequently, my consumption of some of these sweets reduced without any conscious mandate to do so. Meanwhile, my intake of healthier alternatives increased.

Food	Partial List of Ingredients
Chocolate Chip Cookies	3½ Cups of Flour 1 Cup of Butter 1 Cup of White Sugar ¾ Cup of Brown Sugar 1¼ Cup of Chocolate Chips
Shortbread Cookies	1½ Cup of Flour 1 Cup of Butter ½ Cup of Icing Sugar
Blueberry Muffins	2 Cups of Flour ½ Cup of Vegetable Oil ¾ Cup of Brown Sugar 1 Cup of Blueberries
Cheesecake	2 Cups of Cream Cheese 1½ Cup of Sugar ½ Cup of Heavy Cream 4 Eggs
Flourless Chocolate Cake	1½ Cup of Chocolate Chips 1½ Cup of White Sugar 1 Cup of Butter 6 Eggs

Challenging Assumptions

In the old days, it wasn't unusual for me to dive my hand into the box of granola bars three or four times in an evening. The perception I had was that because they were considered healthy, it was safe to eat them indiscriminately.

Little did I realize that consuming two of the chocolate dipped granola bars was tantamount to eating a classic chocolate bar – both in terms of calories and sugar content.

Occasionally I would buy a bag of bagels. Thinking it was no different than any other bread product, I would eat a few. Each large bagel, however, had the same number of calories as four slices of white bread. That's before any thought of cream cheese, which could have doubled that figure.

These foods weren't bad in themselves, but my incorrect assumptions about them led me to consume far more calories than I thought I was taking in.

I've discussed the importance of becoming aware of what was going into my body. Part of that was also to note my predisposition to over-eat foods I classified as healthy.

I found that keeping a food journal was a particularly useful tool in uncovering those internal biases.

Food	Calories
Granola Bar	160
Bagel	360
Fruit Smoothie	550
Yoghurt Parfait	300
Bran Muffin	410
Dried Fruit (¾ Cup)	420
Peanuts (¾ Cup)	810

Cheat Days

I don't do cheat days, though this wasn't always the case. Early on in my journey, I'd cheat once or twice a week. Without fail, I'd feel terrible afterwards. I had worked so hard to shave off a hundred calories over the course of a week, and yet here I had piled on an extra thousand in one day. And I'd keep doing it.

This urge that fuelled cheat days indicated that my approach with my eating as it stood then was untenable. When I asked myself *why* I had consumed so much, I realized it was because I felt that I was missing out on food. So much so that I would make up for the deficiency in short destructive bursts. Without noticing it, I had come to view my weight loss as a chore. I was sure to abandon my attempt if things didn't change.

Once I understood why I cheated, I came up with strategies to address its cause. For instance, I found a way to handle my need to binge (*Managing Binging*, page 48) and a method to enjoy calorie sinks like pizza (*Proportioning Meals*, page 37).

Since coming up with these coping mechanisms, I haven't felt the need to cheat. Sure, there were days where I greatly exceeded my recommended caloric intake. So what? The point is that it was not a frequent event brought on because of a systemic feeling of food being denied.

Bad Days

In my yo-yo diet days, I would punish myself if I thought I had consumed too many calories. Usually, this meant starving myself in a misguided attempt to undo the damage. I've since stopped this destructive pattern.

There's a few reasons for this change of heart. The most vain would be that I would only make myself liable to over-eat once I finally did come into contact with food, risking more excesses. The better explanation was that this was an opportunity to learn.

Whenever I had a bad day, I asked myself what was behind the excess, and what I could do to mitigate it next time. Sometimes, the problem would be as simple as being unaware of how many calories there was in consuming eight chocolate wafer cookies. Solutions might then to look at nutritional labels before eating cookies to get an idea of the cost. If it was high in calories, I might then limit myself to two cookies, and substitute the rest of the cookies with a second less-expensive snack to satisfy the hunger.

Other times, the causes were more complex and less easy to address, such as eating too much at a family meal. I eventually came up with a series of tactics that would help there too (*Family Meals* page 63).

In all cases, there was one or many causes, and something to learn from it. I would glean what I could from the experience and move on.

Skipping Meals

One of the many diets I tried long ago involved restricting myself to eating one large meal a day. Typically it was in the form of a lunch from a restaurant around the corner from where I worked. It was unhealthy, not only because the meal itself usually involved lots of gravy and fried products, but because I was starving myself.

The effects of the measures lasted only as long as the diet itself. Once I stopped, I gained back all the weight I had lost and then some.

I don't restrict myself to a lone meal, nor seek to skip breakfast or any other meals of my day. The idea of starving oneself is neither enjoyable nor sustainable, and deserves all the derision I give to fad diets (*Fad Diets Suck,* page 9).

If another reason is needed to object to the concept of skipping meals, it is that a person is liable to ingest more calories than they would have averted once they finally do eat. So if I skip breakfast, I'll probably be famished come lunch-time, and I risk over-eating.

Finding Motivation

It helped that I wasn't the only one I knew trying to lose weight. A few coworkers and friends were also on their own journeys, and I found their progress truly inspiring. The success they had achieved was confirmation that I too could pull this off.

I also found motivation from within by tapping into my inner-competitive self. I would look at my completed food journal entry for the day, and figure out ways to could reduce the number of total calories without cutting out the things I liked or feeling hungry. I made it into a game that I repeated every day, trying to meter out savings here or there without compromising my love of food.

Exercise

Eating well and exercise are key to leading a healthy life. It's a hard truth whose denial is capitalized upon by the fad diet industry. Yet I have not discussed exercise in this book.

The reason for its absence is simple. In terms of pure weight loss, altering my eating habits was far more influential than getting into shape.

After all, there's as many calories saved by opting to forgo the chocolate bar as there are burned by riding a bicycle for an hour. It takes much less effort to eat something else than to devote an hour of time to an activity.

I could walk for an hour... or skip the soda.

I could bike for an hour... or skip the chocolate bar.

I could jog for an hour... or skip the muffin.

That said, eating better does not excuse an avoidance of exercise. Epidemiologists are clear on this point: both are essential to healthy living.

It's About Being Sensible

Absent from these pages is the demand to weight in. Scales are a double-edged sword. On the one side, when I stepped on the scale and saw that I lost weight, I was imbued with a boost of motivation that helped me continue. After all, though I tried to reduce the footprint the changes to my eating habits were incurring in my life, it still wasn't easy. No change is.

The scale gave recognition of a difficult journey imperceptible to others. On the other hand, I became bonded to its readings in an unhealthy way, as if its numbers decided how good I should feel about myself. Too easily I became depressed if its numbers incremented ever-so-slightly.

I needed to remind myself that this wasn't about being thin, it was about being healthy. Despite much advancement in this regard, abetted with a good dose of therapy, I sometimes lose sight of this.

When I do weigh in, I do not compare the results of one day to another. I look at long term trends, usually over a period of a week. A spreadsheet program can be very useful for this task. My daily weight fluctuations are meaningless otherwise, having much more to do with how hydrated I am than whether I'm losing weight.

Keeping on the theme of being sensible, I hope that by now it's become clear that none of the changes I made on this weight loss journey were drastic. Small changes to my eating choices, a refusal to let myself go hungry, no skipping meals or punishing myself for bad days. Just a slow progression to a better lifestyle.

Strategies

Hungry? Eat!

None of the strategies outlined on the following pages involve food deprivation. If I felt like I was missing out on food or allowed myself to feel hungry, I'd be miserable and sure to abandon the weight loss effort.

Some of the strategies are as simple as making different choices when doing a grocery run (*Grocery Shopping*, page 50) or having healthier snacks more readily available (*Snacking*, page 41). Other tactics may require slightly more mental effort, at least initially, such as making sure to stay hydrated (*Between Meals and Snacks*, page 44).

Never were there any demands to forego the foods I enjoyed. If I wanted that doughnut, I ate that doughnut. Simple as that.

Meal Time

A number of tricks helped to reduce how much I ate during meals. None of them involving telling myself to not eat what I wanted.

Use Small Plates: Having smaller plates encourages the use of smaller portions from the onset. Though I never told myself I couldn't go back for seconds, I would often realize come the end of the first plate that I was in fact satiated. Or that if I did go back, I didn't want as much. Having those smaller plates let me evaluate how full I was sooner.

Eat Slowly: It takes twenty minutes from the time that one is full to actually realizing it. Eating slow lets my mind catch up with my gut, but also lets me better appreciate each bite rather than trying to gulp it all down as if it were a race. This moderates my consumption. I don't put my fork down between each bite or any of that business.

Finish Each Bite: I don't pile on a whole bunch of food on my fork at once, or take another forkful until what is in my mouth is chewed and swallowed. This lets me better appreciate each bite and slow my eating down, making me feel satisfied sooner.

Drink During Meals: While drinking during the meal doesn't contribute to how full I feel overall, it has the effect of slowing down my ingestion of food. If I'm at a restaurant, I always order water with my meal, even if I also have a beer or glass of wine.

Avoid Distractions: I try not to eat main meals in front of the television or computer. When I'm distracted like that, I'm less aware of the food that I'm ingesting, and so more likely to eat more without knowing it.

Get Up To Get More: When I sit down to eat, I don't keep bowls or plates with the rest of the food within reach – healthy items like salads aside. If I want more, I need to get up and get it from the kitchen counter. Having this simple extra step inhibits me from just mindlessly picking off food, which I'm liable to do given that I find it hard to resist what's laid out in front of me.

Have Dedicated Meal Times: I have this tendency to want to eat my lunches and suppers early. I stave off these urges by snacking or having a small meal instead. If I were to indulge in a full-blown meal, then I'd be stuck later in the day with no main dish in sight, and more likely to eat more heavily to make up for the deficit.

Use Small Spoons: Whether for cereal, soup, or ice cream, I always try to use the small spoon. This forces me to take more dips as compared to larger utensils, which drags out the meal and gives me the impression of having eaten more.

Serve Half at a Time: This is especially useful for desserts, but I also do it for some meal items like slices of pizza. If I have a high calorie item, I'll give myself half of what I wanted, with the full intent of going back for the rest. So if I wanted a big slice of cheesecake, I'll cut that in half and put the first half on my plate, and go back for the second half after I'm done.

Had I given myself that big slice of cheesecake on the outset, I might have gone for another big piece. I'm less likely to do that when I've already had two, albeit smaller, slices. Furthermore, if I do go for another slice, it's easier to make it the half-size when that's what I've been giving myself all along.

Proportioning Meals

In addition to the behavioural changes discussed in *Meal Time*, I did learn some tricks to reduce the caloric impact of meals through very subtle changes when preparing food.

2+ Items Rule: Typically my suppers will consist of two or three items. There will be the big ticket item, such as one of my fancy attempts at Chicken Cordon Bleu, and sides such as steamed vegetables and home-made chips.

The big-ticket item is the reason why I'm enjoying the meal. But that does not mean that it needs to dominate in terms of proportions. In fact, I found that slightly reducing the portion of the main item while increasing the amount of less-calorie intensive sides did not have a noticeable impact on my enjoyment of the meal. There were, however, very real savings in the calorie total of the plate.

For foods that don't traditionally have sides, such as spaghetti, I started to add them in. I'd reduce the portion for the main item accordingly. Even though the variety on my plate went up, the calories dropped.

Add Vegetables: Adding vegetables is another way to reduce the calorie count of a number of dishes, particularly those served in bowls. From chili dishes, to pasta sauces, to potato salads – I would add copious amounts of vegetables wherever I could. The meal would taste just as pleasant, but the amount of calories in each bite was reduced.

Fill the Plate with Less: I noticed that an important part of how satisfied I was with a meal had to do with how much area on the plate was taken up by food. Thus if I could make the plate look full with smaller portions, I'd eat less without actually feeling like I was missing out.

For instance, if I was making my own pizza dough, I'd make the crust thinner. The resulting slices wouldn't look any smaller on my plate, and so I didn't feel like anything was amiss when I ate them.

 If I'd make home-made chips to go with my fish, I'd slice the potatoes into really fine wedges. These wedges took the same amount of space on my plate, but they had fewer calories than their thicker predecessors. If I had a chicken breast, I'd cut it, fold it open like a book, and then only put the half on my plate. I found myself just as satiated as the days of eating the whole breast.

I discovered that I could get away with putting half the meat in a wrap as long as I bumped up the vegetable count to make it look as voluminous as before. Rare was the taste or how full I felt impacted, and where it was, I simply reverted to the portions of old.

Bloat It Up: It's tempting to go for a seconds if the original item didn't feel like it was all that substantive. When I made my own burgers for supper, or my own sandwiches for lunch, it wasn't uncommon of me to make two of them. That was twice the bread, twice the high-calorie patties or roast beef.

That changed when I started bloat up the original item. I would make a massive burger – filling it up with lettuce, nearly a whole tomato, cooked onions, and mushrooms. After finishing that, I wasn't nearly as enticed at the prospect of a second. Those fillings meanwhile only incremented the calorie value of the burger by a fraction.

Satiate First

Let's say that I'm hungry and really in the mood for something that's not particularly healthy such as doughnuts.

What I'll try to do is deal with the hunger first, and then address my desire for a particular food. So in the case of the doughnuts, I'll drink some water and snack on something healthier. Then I'll go out and enjoy the pastry.

This is similar logic to the *2+ Item Rule* I have when making meals. There's the main item, the chicken provolone or the lasagna, that is the attraction for the plate. Then there are the sides used to tone down the calorie concentration of the meal.

The end result is that satiating myself first lowers my chances of going back for more of the unhealthy item as a means to satisfy an otherwise empty stomach. I use this trick for dealing with croissants and other morning treats by supplementing them with cereal. Similarly, I address desserts by preceeding them with a satisfying meal.

Snacking

Whether it's at home or at work, snacking is an essential component of my life. Like eating meals, I've come to adopt a number of tricks to help reduce its caloric footprint.

Buy Healthier Snacks: This one tip is the most responsible for reducing the calories I consume by the thousands over a period of a week. Simply said, the easiest way to avoid eating those deadly sandwich cookies is by not buying them in the first place. Instead, I'll buy healthier alternatives such as sugary cereals, fruits, and vegetables conducive to eating as finger food. If I really do want those sandwich cookies, I'll buy the smallest package they have, or buy it with less frequency.

Keep Snacks Out of Hand's Reach: If I want to have a snack, I need to get up and get it. I don't keep it within reach of my sitting position. This is as true at work as it is at home. Otherwise, I'll be much more likely to mindlessly pick away at the food.

Out of Sight is Out of Mind: If I keep seeing that box of cookies on the kitchen counter, I'll be much more likely to want a cookie than if that same box was hidden away in a cupboard. By keeping particularly unhealthy snacks out of sight, I reduce the frequency of which I notice them and therefore consider eating them.

Make Healthy Snacks Accessible: Following on the previous point, I place things in my apartment so that it's more convenient for me to grab vegetables and sugary cereals as snacks than it is to grab chips and cookies. The latter usually involves a stool to get to.

Use Smaller Bowls: If I'm eating pretzels or other finger foods that necessitate the need of a container, I'll dump them into a small bowl. I don't set limits on how many time I can fill that bowl back up, but having to get up to get more is another minor obstacle between me and food. Having those obstacles makes me question whether I actually want more, something which wouldn't concern me if the food was right there in front of me.

Don't Eat Out of the Bag: Chips are particularly bad for this. If I buy a large bag and eat out of it, the completionist in me will find it too easy to keep grabbing more from it until I make my way to the bottom. So I pour out the contents of the bag in a small bowl and eat from that.

Don't Stack: It's tempting to want to grab a handful of nuts or popcorn and put it in my mouth all at once. By instead habituating myself to grabbing one piece at a time, I drag out the time it takes to eat, and I end up feeling like I had more food than I did.

Cut It Up: Where the snack food comes in large items, I'll cut it up into small discrete pieces. With cucumbers, I'll make really thin slices. With carrots, I'll cut it in two or three pieces. In both the previous examples, the end product retains a sense of size, but it takes more time to go through it all. I find that I end up eating less this way, without feeling any less full.

Dip Not Scoop: I used to have a tendency to dunk tortillas into salsa, or vegetables into dip, with the intent of scooping up as much of the tasty sauce as possible. Each single scoop exploded the calorie count of whatever I was eating. I now dip instead of scoop, still giving the same enjoyable taste without packing so many calories. There are times where I'll scoop up, but it's not every single dunk.

Bring Snacks to Work or School: My workplace has a vending machine filled with chocolate bars and bags of chips. If I'm hit with a sudden pang for food while I'm there, I'm liable to make buy one of those items. So I bring plenty of snacks from home to keep me satisfied throughout the day. It's less expensive and easily shaves calories.

Consider a Meal: I always feel much more satisfied after eating a hearty meal than after consuming a snack. Yet, there are times where I'll snack and snack, and the amount of calories I'll have taken in through these snacks will exceed any meal I could have conjured. When I'm particularly famished, I'll ask myself whether I'd be better served by eating a small meal like a bowl of cereal or a sandwich rather than a snack.

Between Meals and Snacks

I also adopted a few strategies outside of the time I devoted to eating that helped with my weight loss.

Sleep Well: A number of studies have found a connection between sleeping well and weight. Cited reasons include slower metabolism when sleep-deprived as well as changes in the hormones that regulate the desire for food. Sleeping at a decent hour also reduces the odds of a late-night snack.

Stay Hydrated: Much of why I eat during the day has to do with yearning for something in my mouth, and not really hunger. I find that drinking water and tea throughout the day addresses this need without adding calories. I don't drink juices except on occasion; I view them as sugar-water with no nutritional value.

Forecast Calories: Before a snack or meal, I'll mentally estimate how many calories are contained. This is to avoid surprises come time to write in the food journal. It also affects my subsequent decision making process.

I don't tell myself that a food is off-limits because there may be lots of calories. If it's a snack, I might instead vary up their contents. Rather than just nuts, I might go for nuts and something else to offset the high calorie content of the former. Or for meals, I'll stick to two portions of chicken instead of three, but bump up the size of the sides. For restaurants, it might make me skip the appetizer in favour of a more satisfying meal with dessert. I become empowered to make small decisions ahead of time so that I feel better about myself afterwards.

Beverages

Drinks aren't usually thought of as being significant, but they can make as much of an impact as food. I've come to increase my intake of water while cutting down on juice, beer, and other high-calories beverages.

Quench Thirst First: After a hot summer day, I like to come home and enjoy a nice cool beer. However, I always precede that by grabbing some water to address my thirst. By dealing with that first, I don't end up mindlessly drinking a bunch of beer.

Always Have Water: Even if I order a beer or wine with my meal at a restaurant, I'll ask for a glass of water as well. I'll consequently come to drink less of the alcohol without feeling any less satiated.

Use Tall Glasses: The glass on the right in the following diagram has 30% more liquid as the one to the left. That this isn't immediately apparent is quite normal.

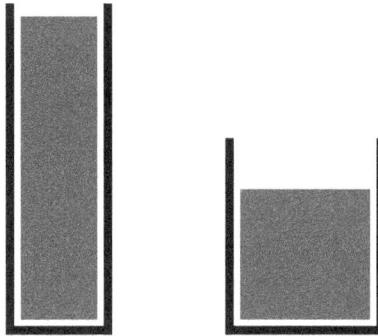

I use tall glasses whenever I serve myself wine or juice. It turns the optical illusion in my favour, making me drink less than when consuming from a stubbier vessel.

Choose Bottles Over Pints: An imperial pint holds 569 millilitres of beer. A Canadian beer bottle by comparison holds 341 millilitres, or about 40% less. Yet I don't find one to be any less satisfying than the other. Consequently, I usually order bottles over pints. It's an easy way to drink less and shave a hundred calories or more.

Reduce Servings of Powdered Mixes: I find that I can cut down a third of the recommended serving of a powdered mix such as hot chocolate without any impact on taste. Since the average mix is almost entirely sugar, the slight reduction does make a difference.

Know What's in the Coffee: A cup of coffee contains five calories. Adding two creams and a tablespoon of sugar makes that figure jump to a hundred calories. While this is still relatively low, having two or three cups of that a day can quickly pile on the calories. I've come to substitute cream for skim milk, decrease my coffee dependence, and up my tea intake.

Managing Binging

Binging is defined as uncontrollable over-eating that can lead to hundreds or thousands of calories being ingested in one sitting. Sometimes it's preceded by an intense feeling of hunger while other times it can be less conscious – such as when I would eat a whole bag of chips while watching a movie at home.

Inextricably linked with the uncontrollable eating was the mixture of regret and disgust that would inevitably follow. I hated myself for binging, but I didn't feel there was anything I could do about it. I was wrong.

Shown in the following picture are two plates. In the plate on the left is a single sandwich cookie. The plate on the right is brimming with vegetables. The platter of greens has fewer calories than the lone cookie, despite being many times as voluminous. When it comes to binging, knowing how to get full on as few calories as possible is critical.

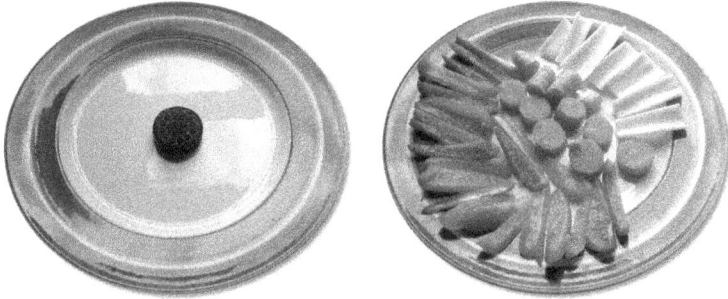

Carrots, celery, apples and oranges are all easy to reach snacks that require no preparation. I made sure that they were always easier to reach than the less healthy options in my house. For binging, I favoured vegetables over fruits because of the lower calorie count of the former.

In cases where I had a crave for a specific food, I'd eat something else first *(Satiate First,* page 40) and if it was finger food, I made an effort to avoid grabbing handfuls of the item at once.

Grocery Shopping

One of the easiest ways I managed to reduce my caloric intake over the course of a week was by changing what I bought while grocery shopping. It can be assumed that I ate what I purchased, so if I bought lots of unhealthy sugary items, those would invariable end up in my food journal.

I greatly increased the amount of vegetables I bought. Every week I'd grab celery, carrots, peppers, broccoli, lettuce, tomatoes and onions. This also fed into my desire to not waste food, which meant that I made more salads so that I didn't end up with bad lettuce, and my other meals contained more vegetables at the expense of less healthy alternatives.

I relegated sugar-pumped children's cereals to the role of snack food and bought toasted oats for my breakfasts. I bought more fish, chicken breasts and steak. Meanwhile, I cut down on breaded fish sticks and other meal items that came in boxes from the frozen food section. Bacon became turkey bacon. Milk became unsweetened almond milk. Mayonnaise became mustard. I switched to lower calorie salad dressings.

I started to make more of my own foods. Instead of buying fries, I bought sweet potatoes which I would cut up at home and lightly oil. Rather than getting ice cream, I obtained molds to make freezer pops from juice.

I bought the ingredients to make my own pies, cakes, and cookies rather than purchasing them ready-to-eat. This extra effort of having to make my own stuff had a few advantages. I would bake and eat the items because I wanted them, not because it was already around to just pick at. Also, I knew what ingredients went in, improving my awareness (*Culinary Exploration*, page 17).

I also used my culinary streak to invest in a bread maker and pasta machine. I would cut up slices of bread for my sandwiches that were half the thickness of their store-bought counterparts, though no less satisfying. I also used the bread maker to make my own pizza dough. With the pasta machine, I made my own lasagnas and vermicelli. Though it sounds like it would take much more time to do all of this, it wasn't all that substantive. The bread maker took no more than a few minutes to throw the ingredients in and the machine did the rest.

I stopped buying pop, chips, and granola bars. Henceforth, I'd have to make a special run to the corner store if I wanted junk food. In the summer, I'd buy watermelons and go to the local farmer's market to pick up in-season fruits and vegetables.

There's a few misconceptions about shopping healthy. The first is that it costs more. I don't agree with this at all. Root vegetables are often the cheapest items per unit pound one can get at a grocery store. Meat from the butcher is also cheaper by weight than its breaded counterpart found in the frozen food aisle. Shopping at discount and bulk food stores yield further savings.

When I lived below the poverty line as a student, I stuck to cheap large bags of frozen vegetables. Nevertheless, had I just invested a third of the money spent for a night of alcohol abuse, cost-saving measures such as pre-drinking included, I could have eaten very well.

Perverting Salads and Other Healthy Foods

Salads are nutritious and have few calories. However, if I dump a whole heap of Caesar dressing on it, the amount of calories it will have jumps through the roof. The same can be said of other foods such as peanut butter applied to celery, cheese spreads to toast, and condiments to sandwiches. There can be more calories in the condiment or sauce than the very food it's meant to embellish.

This is not to say that I don't enjoy dressing with my salad, but I've become more careful with what I add and how much of it I put on. Having this awareness helps me make choices such as being more conservative with how much dip I put on my chips, or favouring mustard over mayonnaise when I make my sandwiches for work. The savings add up.

DIETS SUCK!

Food	Calories
Celery Stalk	10
Celery Stalk with Peanut Butter	180
Garden Salad	70
Garden Salad with Ranch Dressing	300
Sandwich with Mustard	220
Sandwich with Mayo & Cheese	390
Assorted Vegetables	60
Assorted Vegetables with Dip	580
Tofu	90
Fried Tofu	350
Potato Chips	250
Potato Chips with Dip	600

Food in the Age of Plenty

One of the most difficult lessons in this weight-loss journey was coming to grasp with the fact that I didn't need to finish my plate. This went counter to years of conditioning in my youth with messages of starving children in some far off land.

When I wasn't able to serve myself, such as at restaurants and family meals, the portions were far too generous. The completionist in me used to finish off the plate, regardless of how satiated I actually was. Only when I was seemingly bursting at the seems would I stop.

These days, when I'm at a sit-down restaurant, I'll usually eat a good chunk of everything, but there will be left-overs. I make an effort to eat until I'm satiated, not until I'm sick. I won't go for appetizer, as a main course is more than enough in its own right. I have a different approach for buffets (*Buffets*, page 69).

Where the option is there, I'll just order the small size: the six-inch submarine sandwich; the small fries; the small popcorn; the small ice cream cone. The word *small* conjures notions of insufficiency, but the truth is that that's rarely the case – and when it is, I'll go for the size up. In most instances, however, I'll feel satiated on a small wrap than I would its super-sized brethren.

Continuing with the theme, just because it's there doesn't mean I have to eat it. I often make cookies at home, and with that comes the temptation of dip my fingers into the left-over dough that wouldn't make it into the oven. I have this sentiment that it would go to waste otherwise. It's very easy to eat a few cookie's worth of dough just by this flawed idea. To overcome it, I promise myself two cookies after they're done baking. That's still less than eating dough and cookies.

Likewise, when I cook for others, I have this temptation to want to eat the left overs. As if pitching them in the trash meant the food was wasted. I have to remember that I ate until I was satiated and so the food fulfilled its purpose. It's okay to throw it away. Those calories I save just by sticking to what I wanted to eat in the first place add up over time.

We live in an age of plenty, where the excuse that all shreds of food need to be conserved regardless of their usefulness has withered away. If I'm hungry, I'll eat. If I'm not, I shouldn't consume out of a flawed sense of waste.

Dependence on Restaurants

There are two main reasons why I go to restaurants: either because I want to and enjoy a nice meal or socialize, or because I didn't have time to make a proper meal for myself. I try to reduce instances of the latter.

For breakfast, I always make sure that milk and cereal are at my disposal. That eliminates most trips to the greasy spoon around the corner from my office.

For lunch, I'll make sandwiches the day before if I know I'll be in a rush the morning after. Otherwise I try to keep bread and deli meat stocked in the fridge so that making lunches only takes a few minutes. I also have lots of empty plastic containers at the ready to turn one night's left overs into the following day's lunch.

For suppers, there are times where I'm just feeling lazy. In those cases, I'll steam vegetables (few minutes in the microwave) and boil up some pasta. Or I'll go to the grocery store and pick up one of those ready-to-eat barbecued chickens.

I still go to restaurants, but the point is that I try to make it so that it's because I *want* to be there, not because I *have* to be there.

Food Journal Revisited

I ended the previous section with the premise that it was about being sensible. This also meant that a food journal couldn't become a permanent fixture of my life.

The purpose of the journal was to become aware of what impact my eating habits were having and to provide me with insights I could use to reduce my calorie intake.

It was not intended to have me lead a life where I would forever concern myself with how many calories each meal or snack contained. That was the whole point of finding out my sore points and coming up with strategies; so that I could keep my calorie intake in check without thinking about it.

I severed my ties to the food journal about a year into the weight loss journey. I still read the nutritional labels on the packaging of unfamiliar products, but the days of noting the caloric footprint of each foodstuff are over.

Situations

Family Meals

I have a mother who cooks these wonderful five course meals, replete with two or three desserts. Just one of these plates is enough to be a full-blown meal.

The most important thing I keep in mind is that despite what I was taught as a child, I don't have to finish what's before me. If the opportunity is there, I'll serve myself. Otherwise, I'll usually eat less than half of what I was given.

There's also a tendency to follow what others do. So if a few others at the table grab a second helping of potato salad, I might be tempted to do the same – even though I wouldn't have considered that second portion were I alone.

To counter this mob mentality, I'll eat slower than the others as to still have food left when they go for additional helpings. I'll also try to leave a bit on my plate, reducing the amount of times others offer me additional servings. This in turn drops the number of opportunities for me to accept.

I'll also use the same strategies I normally apply to meals at home, such as drinking lots of water and chatting with people (*Meal Time*, page 34).

I won't starve myself as to make room for the impending family meal. I find allowing myself to go hungry makes me liable to over-eat come time to sit at the table, which is probably the worst thing I could do.

Work and School

My work place is characterized by having two vending machines and being in close proximity to three greasy spoons. There's also free doughnuts every Friday and a monthly company barbecue in the summer.

I try to keep the trips to the restaurant at a minimum. I also bring my own snacks to work with me to curb my relationship with the vending machine. Instead of frequently grabbing soft drinks, I began to drink a variety of teas. Just dropping one soda every few days was enough to make me shed a few pounds over the course of a month.

As for the Friday morning pastries, I looked up what was in the selection. I was surprised to discover that muffins were in fact the least healthy option, having typically 450 calories each. I soon stopped grabbing two of them in my mornings. These days, I usually favour the jelly-filled Boston Cream doughnuts. Incidentally, it contains half the calories of the muffin.

The barbecues were a bit more tricky. Had there only been one big-ticket item available, such as say hamburgers, I would have been content with just that. But since there were sausages and chicken as well, I felt like I was missing out if I just stuck to the one meat. The paradox of variety. In the old days, I'd have a hamburger and sausage, both with buns and condiments, plus the chicken. Then there'd be pasta and chips as sides. A single plateful could easily contained my recommended daily caloric intake.

Fast forward to today, and I still have the hamburger with condiments. If I feel like sausage, I'll take a sliver and forgo its bun. Really what I want is a taste of it, not the whole thing. The first bite is great, but I'm indifferent after the third bite. For the sides, I've switched to garden salad, of which there's always a surplus at these events.

I don't leave my lunch or snacks in sight at my desk. I find that I'm much more likely to eat it all early in the morning if I'm constantly reminded of its presence. I put it out of sight, and consequently only grab them when the need arises.

Fast Food

What makes fast food so calorie rich isn't so much the main item, like a burger, but the sides that accompany it. Whereas a burger may be anywhere from 300-600 calories, adding fries and a drink can double to triple that amount.

When I go to a fast food joint, I'll typically go for a burger of a satisfying size, skip the soft drink and perhaps get the small fries. With places that specialize in submarine sandwiches, I'll go for the small wrap (usually six inches), and stock it full of vegetables. I favour lower calorie condiments such as mustard over richer alternatives such as mayonnaise. Having a whole bunch of vegetables makes it more filling and avoids the urge for a side such as cookies.

The issue I find with most other fast food restaurants are the huge portions they give: the big noodle dishes of the Thai place; the massive portions of the Greek shop. Though I'm tempted to eat all that is before me, I find that I'm just as satisfied if I stop at the halfway mark. As for the left-overs, I'll usually pitch them. The reason being that they never end up lasting until the next day as I would like.

Instead, the extras get eaten as they linger on my work desk, or on the bus ride home, or as I walk in through the front door. It's very hard to resist food from a fast food place when it's within reach. So I dispose of them.

Contrary to the consumerist instinct, this isn't throwing money down the drain. I got what I paid for: a satisfying meal.

The most difficult part of my association with fast food was to overcome my aversion to items labelled *small*. I had this idea that small meant insufficient. It didn't help that the size up was called *regular* or *medium*, implying that the smaller size was outside the norm.

I've come to find that with near universality, small actually means *the right portions*, medium implies *too much*, large signifies *way too much*, and extra large means *lethal*. In some cases, such as the popcorn served at the cinema, even the small bag could be considered *too much*.

Food	Calories
Cheeseburger	300
Deluxe Burger	560
Cheeseburger with Fries & Soft Drink	1180
Submarine Sandwich	350
Submarine Sandwich with 2 Cookies	790
Submarine Sandwich with Soup	440

Buffets

I love buffets. There's a particularly good restaurant near my apartment that has tables upon tables of delicious international selection. In previous times, these establishments were also places where I would eat way too much. I'd fill a plate to the brim and keep eating until I was well beyond the point of stuffed.

These days, I still go to buffets, though I've adopted a few tactics to prevent the kind of abuses that characterized my past trips. Chiefly, I don't pile items on top of each other. I make sure that vegetables are well represented. To deal with the temptation of variety, I'll have a regular-sized portion of one high-calorie item, and tiny portions for the others. These give me satisfying bites. I limit myself to about five items per plate, with each getting its own dedicated area.

Part of my abuse of buffets came from the fact that I didn't feel like I got my money's worth if I didn't go back for seconds or thirds. I've since shed this mentality, realizing that my stomach is quite content with a single dinner and dessert plate. After all, it is my gut that should dictate how much I eat, not my wallet.

I don't forbid myself from seconds, but rare is the time I'll find the need to indulge. I feel just as satiated as those days of piling spoonfuls onto my plate, minus the terrible pains in my stomach.

As usual, I also employ the general tactics that I apply to all meals, such as eating slow and drinking lots of water (*Meal Time*, page 34).

Public Houses

Pubs are one of those places where calories can just pile up. A pint of my favourite maritime ale has 280 calories. A Caesar, the popular Canadian cocktail that mixes vodka, tomato-clam juice, and Worcestershire sauce has about 170. Rare is the time that I have but one of these beverages. And so it was that the calories in the drinks accompanying my meals often exceeded that of the meal itself.

I've made a few changes to my consumption habits. I order beers from bottles instead of pints. It's a smaller vessel, and so fewer calories, but no less satisfying than a pint. I typically also go for two beers. The first I drink at a regular pace, to bring on the arguably pleasant effects related to the intake of alcohol.

The second beer bottle is for show. I'll drink it very slowly, and is used to ward off the societal pressures that comes from having everyone else have a beverage on hand. After I'm done the second bottle, I'll switch to tea or coffee. By this point, the pressure to drink has usually gone.

I also always order water with my alcoholic beverage. I'll alternate between drinking it and the cocktail or beer. I don't want to satisfy my thirst with alcohol – that's what water is for.

If I'm planning on eating at the pub, I'll usually grab a bit of food at home beforehand. What I'll have at home will be healthy, typically fruits and vegetables. This is to prevent my showing up at the pub famished, where I might then order an appetizer or over-eat from the calorie-rich meals.

On my late-night walk homes after a stay at the pub, I'm usually quite hungry and tempted to stop by one of the many shawarma joints that litter my city. Yet a single one of their wraps, with its beef and hefty servings of sauces, can rack up a thousand calories. So instead I try to hold off so that I eat at home. Better to have a shawarma because I want to, not because of alcohol-induced urges.

Drink	Calories
Beer (bottle)	170
Beer (pint)	280
Vodka, Rum, or Gin (shot)	100
Vodka and Soda Water	100
Vodka and Pop	180
Wine (glass)	170
Wine (half-bottle)	260

Coffee Shops and Ice Cream Parlours

Coffee doesn't sound like it's that bad on the outset. Neither does a small ice cream cone. This is of course true, both have a low amount of calories.

However, that doesn't mean that all the selection available at one of these places is just as good. While black coffee might have a handful of calories, the calories quickly pile up when adding milk and sugar. Meanwhile, a flavoured latte, with its syrup and steamed milk, could have a few hundred calories.

The story is similar with ice cream parlours. Whereas a small cone might have a few hundred calories, a modest sum for a treat, some of their other selections can exceed a thousand.

I still consume lattes and luxury ice creams. Like any food, moderation is key. What's different now is that instead of having these items regularly, I relegate them to the status of *treat* - something I'll do here and there.

As with so many other things, merely being aware of how many calories are in some of my favourite treats subconsciously impacts my decision making process. It means that more often than not, I'll pick that small cone over the blizzard.

Food	Calories
Black Coffee	5
Coffee (2 Milks, 2 Sugars)	150
Flavoured Latte	250
Mocha	400
Small Ice Cream Cone	230
Sunday	610
Blizzard	1000

Movie Theatre

Popcorn is another of those food items that can be low in calories, but can also greatly exceed expectations in this regard if unaware the impact of adding butter and its portion sizes.

A small bag of unadulterated popcorn will have around 350 calories. Adding butter nearly doubles that count. Going for the bucket can have as much as 1,600 calories. That's nearly the recommended daily caloric intake in a single sitting. Popcorn doesn't usually elicit thoughts of being a calorie sink, in fact, quite the contrary. This is why awareness combined with an appreciation for moderation is so important.

It must be said that I do find it tempting to go for the large everything while at the cinema. It's only a few cents more than their overpriced smaller counterparts, and so there's this feeling of being ripped off if I don't take advantage of the wonky pricing scheme.

Yet when I listen to my stomach, it's satisfied with the small. Oh sure I could easily eat more if more was there to eat, but that's not because there's a genuine desire for more.

That's because it's very hard to resist food when it's laid in front of me. When I walk out of the movie theatre after having had a small popcorn, I'm just as satiated as when I had the large bucket – minus perhaps the feeling of imminent explosion that tends to follow the latter.

Going back to the money argument, the smaller bag is cheaper. It's a win-win. Oh sure, the cost savings are only by a few cents, but it's still a savings. The pricing scheme is purposefully there to inhibit this decision, the result of very clever marketing research. Once I realized that I was in it to feel satiated, not pander to the executives, it became easier to order the small by default.

Food	Calories
Small Popcorn (No Butter)	350
Small Popcorn (Buttered)	630
Bucket of Popcorn (No Butter)	1,100
Bucket of Popcorn (Buttered)	1,600
Small Candy	260
Large Candy	820
Medium Soft Drink	290

Vacations and Work Trips

When I'm away from home, either for work or vacation, I become dependent on restaurants. It's near impossible to avoid.

There's a few strategies I adopt when on these trips. I make an effort not to go to fast food places, favouring the simple sandwiches one can buy at grocery stores. I stick to coffee and tea, relegating soft drinks to the status of treat.

I'll purchase some basic food supplies. Usually vegetables, fruits, snacks, bread and peanut butter – items that don't necessitate a refrigerator and which can be turned into snacks or meals.

In countries where water quality might be an issue, I make sure that anything grown in the ground has a thick peal and isn't cut up. Whole oranges for instance.

I'll also get large bottles of water, typically 1 to 1.5 litres, which will trod around with me. This helps me keep hydrated and avoid the ubiquitous sugary alternatives.

If the food is free, such as at a hotel or resort, I'll be tempted to try everything. Especially if there are lots of delicious-looking pastries and desserts.

To counter this instinct, I limit myself to one or two new of these high-calorie items a day and make sure to fill the rest of my plate with healthier options. I then tell myself to go back to my favourite item on my last day there.

Example Meals

A Note for the Reader

I don't like meal guides. The ingredients listed usually aren't anything I'll have at my fridge or cupboards, they ignore my food preferences, and they don't reflect how much time I have to make it.

Thus, the meals listed on the following pages aren't meant to be a plan to follow. The reason they're included is to illustrate how I can balance a reduced calorie intake while eating the things I enjoy.

Note that in all cases, the total number of calories listed for each day falls below my recommended daily levels. In other words, there's room to add food beyond what's already listed.

Day One

This is a typical day. Note that even though I have less than 2,000 calories, I still managed to fit in a number of treats: a coke, a beer, cheesecake, and a small bag of chips.

Food	Calories
Cereal & Unsweetened Soy Milk	140
Banana	110
Black Coffee	5
Carrot	40
2 x Celery Stalks	20
Sandwich (Roast Beef, Lettuce, Mustard)	210
Soda	160
Chips (Small Bag)	210
Fish Fillet	110
Baked Potato	160
Steamed Vegetables	40
Beer	160
Cheesecake	450
Apple	80
Popcorn (3 Cups)	90

Total: 1,985

Day Two

This day starts off with a solid breakfast involving bacon and eggs and culminates with an evening watching movies while enjoying tortilla chips and salsa.

Food	Calories
Single Egg	70
Turkey Bacon (2 Slices)	60
Buttered Toast (2 Slices)	260
Black Coffee	5
Apple	80
Wrap (½ Burger, Mustard, Vegetables)	260
Orange	70
Sugary Cereal	100
Lemongrass Tea	0
Chicken Breast	260
Garden Salad & Dressing	180
Cold Pasta	180
2 x Cookies	160
Tortilla Chips & Salsa	350

Total: 2,035

Day Three

This third day begins with a bigger-than-usual bowl of cereal to wake me up. I make myself a loaded veggie burger for dinner, filled with nearly an entire tomato, lettuce, green peppers, mushrooms, and mustard. I end the day with raspberry pie and ice cream.

Food	Calories
Cereal & Almond Milk	250
Black Coffee	5
Carrot	40
2 x Celery Stalks	20
Sandwich (Bacon, Lettuce, Tomato)	240
Apple	80
Hot Chocolate	70
Burger	450
Home-made Fries	180
Raspberry Pie	330
Cucumber	30
Orange	70
Ice Cream	200

Total: 1,985

Day Four

This is doughnut day at work. I grab a jelly-filled Boston Cream. I enjoy some left-overs for lunch followed by a nice dinner involving pork and a glass of wine. I skip dessert, opting for two cookies and an ice pop.

Food	Calories
Doughnut	250
Black Coffee	5
Sugary Cereal	80
Left-Over Lasagna	350
Banana	110
2 x Celery Stalks	20
Black Coffee	5
2 x Pork Chops	310
Steamed Vegetables	40
Mashed Yam	200
Wine	170
2 x Cookies	160
Ice Pop	80
Apple	80

Total: 1,860

Day Five

The highlight of this fifth day is a steak dinner that's accompanied by steamed butternut squash, brown rice, and an orange juice cocktail. A cup of tea provides a soothing conclusion to the evening.

Food	Calories
Cereal & Unsweetened Soy Milk	140
Toast with Peanut Butter	250
Black Coffee	5
Carrot	80
2 x Celery Stalks	20
Sandwich (Turkey, Cucumber, Dijon)	220
Garden Salad	100
Apple	80
Sirloin Steak	250
Diced Butternut Squash	250
Brown Rice	125
Screwdriver	180
Nuts	130
Broccoli	50
Celery Stalk	10
Sugary Cereal	100
Cranberry Tea	0

Total: 1,990

Conclusion

My learning process on this journey can be broken up into two stages. The first was to become aware of what I was eating and its cost. A big part of this involved using a food journal to uncover how much I was consuming and why. The second stage was to come up with tricks to reduce that cost without going hungry or depriving myself of the foods I liked.

I came to employ a number of psychological tricks to reduce my intake: smaller plates, keeping food out of sight, the insertion of more checkpoints to re-evaluate how full I was, and adding more obstacles between me and food.

I also began substituting some foods for others, which mitigated the damage done by binging, and tweaking proportions in my meals in ways that were visually imperceptible. All measures added up in the long run into real reductions in weight.

Note that not many of the ideas were my own. A great inspiration was the work of Brian Wansink, author of *Mindless Eating: Why We Eat More Than We Think*. A food psychologist, his research found out how our perceptions can affect our eating habits. I also found value in *The*

Volumetrics Weight-Control Plan by Barbara Rolls and Robert Barnett. Other ideas were born out of reading articles on reputable health websites.

The point in doing all of these subtle changes was that I could never afford for this weight loss to become a chore. If it did, it was no longer sustainable, jeopardizing any chances of keeping off the pounds. That's not to say it wasn't without its challenges, as is expected with any lifestyle change, but it felt fair and doable.

This book is not intended to be a step-by-step guide for others to follow. Weight-loss is a deeply personal process, and there is not a single mold that will fit everyone. The reason these strategies worked for me was precisely because I was the one to choose them. They reflected that I was my own cook, that I had binging issues, that I liked doughnuts, that I wasn't a heavy drinker.

So what's on these pages shouldn't be followed like a script. Rather, it should be seen as a collection of ideas, where the ones that resonate with the reader can extracted and made to work in their own life.

I am not a nutritionist nor a weight loss expert, and this book is certainly not a substitute for consulting a medical professional. What I am is a person that embarked on a journey to lose weight, found success, and put together what I thought made it all work.

www.ingramcontent.com/pod-product-compliance
Lightning Source LLC
Chambersburg PA
CBHW022123280326

41933CB00007B/526